A COMPLETE GUIDE ON DIABETES

The ultimate guide on how to reverse
insulin resistance permanently in type 1,
type 2, prediabetes and gestational diabetes

Angel L. Hager

TYPE OF CONTENT

CHAPTER ONE

INTRODUCTION

Diabetes is a chronic (long-lasting) health disease that affects how your body transforms food into energy. Diabetes is a disease in which there is too much glucose (a form of sugar) in the blood. Over time, excessive blood glucose levels may harm the body's organs. Possible long-term consequences include damage to major (macrovascular) and tiny (microvascular) blood arteries, which may lead to heart attack, stroke, and issues with the kidneys, eyes, mouth, feet and nerves.

Your body breaks down most of the food you consume into sugar (glucose) and releases it into your circulation. When your blood sugar goes high, it tells your pancreas to produce insulin. Insulin operates like a key to allow the blood sugar into your body's cells for usage as energy.

With diabetes, your body doesn't create enough insulin or can't utilize it as effectively as it should. When there isn't enough insulin or cells stop reacting to insulin, too much blood sugar lingers in your system. Over time, it might create major health concerns, such as heart disease, eyesight loss, and renal illness.

The good news is that you may lower the risk of the long-term complications of diabetes by maintaining blood pressure, blood glucose and cholesterol levels within suggested range. Also, having a healthy weight, eating properly, decreasing alcohol consumption, and not smoking can also minimize your risk. Regular check-ups and screening are vital to identify any abnormalities early.

If you have diabetes it's vital to incorporate a broad range of nutritional and healthful meals in your diet, and to avoid snacking on sugary foods.

Enjoy a variety of meals from each food category - be sure to include foods rich in fiber and low in fat and decrease your salt consumption. It's essential to contact with a nutritionist to examine your current eating plan and give a guidance regarding food choices and food portions. Limit alcohol consumption. If you consume alcohol, have no more than two standard drinks each day. If you are pregnant or contemplating pregnancy or are nursing, then zero alcohol consumption is suggested.

Smoking is the largest single lifestyle risk factor for acquiring diabetes problems. Smoking may reverse all the advantages acquired by weight reduction, healthy nutrition, excellent blood glucose and blood pressure management.

Smoking impacts circulation by raising heart rate and blood pressure, and by making tiny blood vessels smaller. Smoking also makes blood cells and blood vessel walls sticky and permits hazardous fatty

material to build up. This may lead to heart attack, stroke and other blood vessel problems.

People with diabetes who smoke have higher blood glucose levels and worse control over their diabetes than non-smokers with diabetes

CAUSE

Insulin is a hormone generated by the pancreas to manage blood sugar. Diabetes may be caused by too little insulin, resistance to insulin, or both.

To comprehend diabetes, it is vital to first understand the typical process by which food is broken down and utilized by the body for energy. Several processes happen when food is digested and absorbed:

- A substance called glucose enters the circulation. Glucose is a source of fuel for the body.
- An organ called the pancreas generates insulin. The purpose of insulin is to transfer glucose from the circulation into muscle, fat, and other cells, where it may be stored or utilized as fuel.

People with diabetes have high blood sugar because their body cannot transport sugar from the blood into muscle and fat cells to be burnt or stored for energy, and/or because their liver creates too much glucose and releases it into the blood. This is because either:

- Their pancreas does not generate enough insulin
- Their cells do not react to insulin properly (also termed insulin resistance)

COMMON SIGNS OF DIABETES ARE:

- being extremely thirsty or hungry
- passing more urine (wee) than usual
- feeling tired
- unexplained weight loss (for type 1 diabetes), or progressive weight gain (for type 2 diabetes)
- having injuries that heal slowly
- itching skin or skin infections
- blurred vision

CHAPTER TWO

TYPES OF DIABETES

Type 1 diabetes mellitus (T1D) is an autoimmune illness that leads to the loss of insulin-producing pancreatic beta cells. There is variation in the metabolic, genetic, and immunogenetic aspects of type 1 diabetes and age-related changes, necessitating a tailored therapy for each individual. Loss of insulin secretion may occur immediately or gradually. Residual insulin production (detectable/higher c-peptide) is more prevalent in adult-onset compared to youth-onset type 1 diabetes , although diabetic ketoacidosis is more common in kids with type 1 diabetes . Detectable c-peptide is related with improved glycemic control The existence of other autoimmune disorders, obesity, comorbidities, and the development of diabetes-related complications is also varied. Successful care of type 1 diabetes needs multiple daily insulin injections (MDI), insulin pump therapy, or the use of an automated insulin delivery system, as well as glucose monitoring, ideally using a continuous glucose monitor (CGM). All patients with type 1 diabetes should be able to undertake capillary blood glucose monitoring (BGM) if CGM is unavailable. Self-management education, training, and support, as well as treating psychological difficulties, assist to maximize results. A collaborative multidisciplinary strategy, including medical providers, nurse and dietitian educators, pharmacists, community resources, and specialists when required (including podiatrists, mental health experts, social workers, ophthalmologists, cardiologists, and others), is advised.

Type 1 diabetes, historically known as juvenile diabetes or insulin-dependent diabetes, is a chronic illness. In this disease, the pancreas generates little or no insulin.

Insulin is a hormone the body uses to enable sugar (glucose) to enter cells to make energy.

Different causes, such as genetics and certain viruses, may cause type 1 diabetes. Although type 1 diabetes commonly starts during infancy or adolescence, it may develop in adulthood.

Even after a lot of study, type 1 diabetes has no treatment. Treatment is geared on managing the quantity of sugar in the blood using insulin, food and lifestyle to avoid problems.
 the number of detectable antibodies and the higher their titers, the greater the chance of developing type 1 diabetes .

EPIDEMIOLOGY

Type Type 1 diabetes is one of the most prevalent chronic disorders in children but may have its beginning at any age. In adults, new-onset type 1 diabetes may be misinterpreted as type 2 diabetes and is more frequent than youth-onset type 1 diabetes .There has been a consistent rise in the incidence and prevalence of type 1 diabetes , representing around 5% to 10% of adults with diabetes. A comprehensive review and meta-analysis found that the global prevalence of type 1 diabetes was 9.5%, with an incidence of 15 per 100,000 persons. Worldwide, there is also a large regional difference in occurrence. The largest documented instances are in Finland and other Northern European countries, with rates nearly 400 times larger than those observed in China and Venezuela, where there is the lowest known frequency.

PATHOPHYSIOLOGY

The development of type 1 diabetes happens in 3 phases.

Stage 1 is asymptomatic and characterized by normal fasting glucose, normal glucose tolerance, and the presence of ≥2 pancreatic autoantibodies.

Stage 2 diagnostic criteria include the presence of pancreatic autoantibodies (typically numerous) and dysglycemia: impaired fasting glucose (fasting glucose 100 to 125 mg/dL) or impaired glucose tolerance (2-hour post-75 gm glucose load glucose 140 to 199 mg/dL) or a HbA1c 5.7% to 6.4%. Individuals stay asymptomatic.

In stage 3, there is diabetes, characterized as hyperglycemia (random glucose ≥200 mg/dL) with clinical symptoms, fasting glucose ≥126 mg/dL, glucose ≥200 mg/dL two hours after swallowing 75 g of glucose during an oral glucose tolerance test and/or HbA1c ≥6.5%. If the person lacks conventional signs of hyperglycemia or hyperglycemic crisis, it is advised that two tests be conducted (simultaneously or at various times) to confirm the diagnosis. If there is an initial start of symptoms with hyperglycemia, as more typically happens with youth-onset type 1 diabetes , HbA1c may be deceptive at the time of diagnosis, and glucose criteria should be employed.

type 1 diabetes , particularly in children, usually manifests with hyperglycemic symptoms, which may be abrupt, and include polydipsia, polyuria, polyphagia, nocturnal enuresis, impaired vision, unintended weight loss, weariness, and weakness. If not assessed and treated immediately, it might become a medical emergency. In addition to hyperglycemia, electrolyte imbalances may be present. If these patients are not treated, DKA may develop, necessitating hospitalization and treatment with IV fluids, insulin, potassium, and careful monitoring. Almost one-third of kids present with DKA.

In adult-onset diabetes, the onset of symptoms is more varied than in adolescence, and DKA is less prevalent. It might be difficult to identify type 1 diabetes from type 2 diabetes. GAD65 should be the first antibody tested when diagnosing type 1 diabetes in adults is suspected. If negative and/or if accessible, IA2 and/or ZNT8 should be assessed as well. C-peptide levels may be utilized when there is a doubt regarding whether kind of diabetes is present. A random C-peptide should be obtained with concomitant serum glucose. If the duration of diabetes exceeds three years, c-peptide >600 pmol/L strongly implies type 2 diabetes. A low (<200 pmol/L) or undetectable c-peptide validates the diagnosis of type 1 diabetes

ROLE OF INSULIN IN HUMAN BODY

Insulin is a hormone that originates from a gland placed below and below the stomach (pancreas).

- The pancreas secretes insulin into the circulation.
- Insulin circulates, enabling sugar to enter your cells.
- Insulin decreases the quantity of sugar in your bloodstream.
- As your blood sugar level lowers, so does the release of insulin from your pancreas.

CAUSES OF DIABETES MELLITUS TYPE 1

The specific causation of type 1 diabetes is uncertain. Most likely it is an autoimmune condition.

- This is a disorder that arises when the immune system erroneously targets and kills healthy bodily tissue.
- With type 1 diabetes, an infection or another trigger prompts the body to wrongly target the cells in the pancreas that create insulin.
- The potential to acquire autoimmune disorders, including type 1 diabetes, may be handed down through families.

Risk FACTORS OF DIABETES MELLITUS TYPE 1

Some known risk factors for type 1 diabetes include:

- Family history. Anyone with a parent or sibling with type 1 diabetes has a slightly greater chance of acquiring the illness.

- The presence of specific genes suggests an increased chance of acquiring type 1 diabetes.
- The incidence of type 1 diabetes tends to grow as you go farther from the equator.
- Although type 1 diabetes may emerge at any age, it appears at two prominent peaks. The first peak occurs in youngsters between 4 and 7 years old, while the second is in children between 10 and 14 years old.

COMPLICATIONS OF DIABETES MELLITUS TYPE 1

Eventually, diabetes complications may be disabling or even life-threatening.

- Heart and blood vessel illness. Diabetes greatly raises your risk of many cardiovascular diseases, including coronary artery disease with chest discomfort (angina), heart attack, stroke, narrowing of the arteries (atherosclerosis) and high blood pressure.

- Nerve injury (neuropathy). Excess sugar may harm the walls of the small blood arteries (capillaries) that supply your nerves, particularly in the legs and finally lose all sensation of feeling in the afflicted limbs.
- Damage to the nerves that influence the gastrointestinal system may cause difficulties with nausea, vomiting, diarrhea or constipation. For males, erectile dysfunction may be a concern. Kidney injury (nephropathy). The kidneys contain millions of small blood artery clusters that filter waste from your blood. Diabetes may harm this sensitive filtration mechanism. Severe damage may lead to renal failure or irreversible end-stage kidney disease, which needs dialysis or a kidney transplant.

- Eye damage. Diabetes may damage the blood vessels of the retina (diabetic retinopathy), possibly causing blindness such as cataracts and glaucoma.
- Foot harm. Nerve injury in the feet or inadequate blood supply to the feet raises the risk of many foot problems. Left untreated, scrapes and blisters may cause dangerous infections that may eventually need toe, foot or limb amputation.
  Skin and mouth issues, Diabetes may make you more vulnerable to infections of the skin and mouth, including bacterial and fungal infections. Gum disease and dry mouth also are more frequent.
- Pregnancy problems. High blood sugar levels may be risky for both the mother and the baby. The risk of miscarriage, stillbirth and birth abnormalities rises when diabetes isn't well-controlled. For the mother,

diabetes raises the risk of diabetic ketoacidosis, diabetic eye issues (retinopathy), pregnancy-induced high blood pressure and preeclampsia.

SIGNS AND SYMPTOMS OF DIABETES MELLITUS TYPE 1

The following symptoms may be the first signs of type 1 diabetes. Or they may occur when blood sugar is high.

- Being very thirsty
- Feeling hungry
- Feeling tired all the time
- Having blurry eyesight
- Feeling numbness or tingling in your feet
- Losing weight without trying
- Urinating more often (including urinating at night or bedwetting in

children who were dry overnight before)

For some individuals, these urgent warning symptoms may be the earliest indicators of type 1 diabetes. Or, they may happen when blood sugar is exceedingly high (diabetic ketoacidosis):

- Deep, rapid breathing
- Dry skin and mouth
- Flushed face
- Fruity breath odor
- Nausea or vomiting; inability to keep down fluids
- Stomach pain

DIAGNOSIS AND TEST FOR DIABETES MELLITUS TYPE 1

- A fasting blood glucose test checks your blood glucose level after 8 hours of fasting (no food or drink, except water). This test is not always trustworthy, and tends to be more accurate in the morning. Multiple tests taken at distinct periods are often necessary for a diabetes diagnosis.

- Oral glucose tolerance test. If your first fasting blood glucose test results are normal, but you have any symptoms or risk factors for diabetes, this test is used to diagnosis. A random blood glucose test analyzes your glucose level at an indeterminate time. A high blood glucose level, in addition to experiencing one or more symptoms of diabetes, might suggest that you have the illness. This test is less accurate than a fasting glucose or oral glucose tolerance test.

- The glycated hemoglobin test, or A1C test, is a new form of blood test that offers an overview of your blood glucose levels throughout the last several months, rather than simply a snapshot of your present level. It quantifies the amount of blood sugar bound to the oxygen-carrying protein in red blood cells (hemoglobin). The greater your blood sugar levels, the more hemoglobin you'll have with sugar attached. An A1C score of 6.5 percent or greater on tw independent tests suggests diabetes.

TREATMENT AND MEDICATIONS OF TYPE 1 DIABETES

Type 1 diabetes begins when your body doesn't create any insulin. This means you'll require frequent insulin therapy to keep your glucose levels acceptable. People with type 1 diabetes consequently need lifelong insulin treatment. Insulin comes in various distinct formulations, each of which operates somewhat differently

TYPE OF INSULIN

There are various distinct forms of insulin, which vary depending on how soon they start functioning, when they peak in activity, and how long they persist.

- Rapid-acting insulin, such as Afrezza, Humalog (insulin lispro), Apidra (insulin glulisine), and Novo Rapid and NovoLog (insulin aspart), starts working about 15 minutes after administration, peaks after about one hour, and continues to work for two to four hours, according to the American Diabetes Association.
- Regular (short-acting) insulin, such as Humulin R and Novolin R, starts working after about 30 minutes, peaks after two to three hours, and continues to work for three to six hours.
- Intermediate-acting insulin, such as NPH insulin (Humulin N and Novolin N), starts working after about two to four hours, peaks after 4 to 12 hours, and continues to work for 12 to 18 hours.

- Long-acting insulin, such as Levemir (insulin detemir) and Lantus or Toujeo (insulin glargine), starts working several hours after delivery and has a fairly steady effect over a 24-hour period.

INSULIN INJECTION INTO PANCREATIC

Insulin cannot be given orally because the stomach's digestive acids would destroy the hormone. It must instead be administered by injection, using an insulin pen or a syringe, or via an insulin pump.

THE INSULIN PEN

This device carries either a cartridge or a prefilled reservoir of insulin which will normally last up to 30 days. It has a very tiny needle and the user may dial the needed dosage of insulin and push to inject it.

THE INSULIN PUMP

An insulin pump is a little pager-sized device which constantly distributes insulin via a small tube sited just beneath the person's skin. Extra insulin may be supplied with meals and/or when the blood glucose level is high.

MEDICATIONS

In addition to insulin, some patients with type 1 diabetes may also take Symlin (pramlintide), an injectable medication that may help control abrupt spikes in blood glucose levels after meals (postprandial hyperglycemia).

Pramlintide works by delaying the pace at which food travels through the stomach, as well as by lowering the liver's glucose synthesis.

Other suggested treatments for type 1 diabetes include:

- GlucaGen (glucagon) to treat low blood glucose induced by insulin treatment
- Drugs for high blood pressure
- Drugs for cholesterol control
- Aspirin for prevention of heart disease
- Life style care for treatment of type 1 diabetes

Certain lifestyle alterations may help patients with type 1 diabetes remain healthy and effectively control their illness. These include:

- Monitoring blood glucose levels by monitoring your glucose many times per day using glucose meters
- Eating a well-balanced diet and monitoring carbohydrate consumption (carbs considerably alter blood glucose levels)

- Regular exercise, which may reduce blood glucose and boost the body's sensitivity to insulin

People with diabetes have an increased chance of having foot issues, because the condition may damage nerves and blood vessels in the feet. This risk may be lowered by by:

- Not smoking
- Checking your feet every day, and receiving routine foot checkups throughout the year
- Treating athlete's foot and other foot infections quickly
- Moisturizing the feet with lotion
- Wearing shoes intended to decrease diabetic foot issues

PREVENTION OF DIABETES MELLITUS TYPE 1

- Immunotherapy: Prevent the start or progression of autoimmune destruction of insulin-producing Beta cells. Block the damaging immunological T cells. Support Regulatory cells which protect against autoimmunity Make a commitment to control your diabetes.
- Identify yourself.Wear a tag or bracelet that states you have diabetes. Keep a glucagon kit available in case of a low blood sugar emergency Schedule an annual physical checkup and frequent eye checks.
- Keep your vaccines up to date.High blood sugar might impair your immune system. Get a flu vaccination every year. Your doctor will likely suggest the pneumonia vaccination, as well.
- Pay attention to your feet.Wash your feet everyday with lukewarm water. Dry them carefully, particularly between the toes. Moisturize your feet

with lotion. Check your feet every day for blisters, cuts, sores, redness or swelling. Consult your doctor if you have a sore or other foot condition that doesn't cure.

- Keep your blood pressure and cholesterol under control. If you smoke or use other kinds of tobacco, contact your doctor to help you stop. Smoking raises the chance of diabetic complications, including heart attack, stroke, nerve damage and kidney failure.

- If you consume alcohol, do it responsibly.Alcohol may induce either high or low blood sugar, depending on how much you drink.

- Take stress seriously.The chemicals your body may release in reaction to extended stress may hinder insulin from functioning correctly, which may stress and upset you even more.

CHAPTER THREE

TYPE 2 DIABETES

Type 2 diabetes, the most prevalent kind of diabetes, is a condition that happens when your blood glucose, sometimes called blood sugar, is too high. Blood glucose is your major source of energy and comes mostly from the food you consume. Insulin, a hormone created by the pancreas, helps glucose flow into your cells to be utilized for energy. In type 2 diabetes, your body doesn't create enough insulin or doesn't utilize insulin properly. Too much glucose therefore lingers in your blood, and not enough reaches your cells.

The good news is that you can take efforts to avoid or postpone the development of type 2 diabetes.

PATHOPHYSIOLOGY

Type 2 diabetes mellitus is typically related with particular genetic predispositions, environmental influences, lifestyle choices, and the dynamic interplay between all of these diverse components. This sickness is a disease condition which includes the malfunction of insulin-producing pancreatic beta cells, insulin hormone resistance in cells of the body, or a combination of both. Diabetes mellitus type 2 is a disorder that often starts with resistance to insulin by cells of the body that develops over time. This resistance, and the compensatory generation of insulin by pancreatic beta cells may ultimately lead to beta cell loss. When the beta cells die, endogenous insulin can no longer be released.

Insulin resistance is the inability of cells to utilize the insulin hormone, which restricts the cell's power to absorb and subsequently use glucose in metabolic activities. This is of significant importance in cells that are normally high in metabolic activity, such as muscle, liver, and adipose tissues. Since insulin is responsible for the cellular absorption of glucose, the sugar molecules will stay in the circulation.

The pancreatic beta cells, which are responsible for making and releasing insulin, may also malfunction in type 2 diabetes mellitus. If the insulin supply drops totally, the person will be reliant upon exogenous insulin.

Whether insulin is not present owing to hyposecretion, or if the hormone is rendered ineffective because of insulin resistance, the final outcome will be hyperglycemia. Hyperglycemia, or high glucose levels within the blood, is the characteristic of type 2 diabetes mellitus. Hyperglycemia, and the related inflammatory processes contribute to the micro and macro-vascular alterations that are recognised as consequences of diabetes mellitus.

You can develop type 2 diabetes at any age, even during childhood. However, type 2 diabetes occurs most often in middle-aged and older people. You are more likely to develop type 2 diabetes if you are age 45 or older, have a family history of diabetes, or are overweight or have obesity. Diabetes is more common in people who are African American, Hispanic/Latino, American Indian, Asian American, or Pacific Islander.

Physical inactivity and certain health problems such as high blood pressure affect your chances of developing type 2 diabetes. You are also more likely to develop type 2 diabetes if you have prediabetes or had gestational diabetes when you were pregnant.

SYMPTOMS OF TYPE 2 DIABETES

Symptoms of type 2 diabetes include increased thirst and urination increased hunger feeling tired blurred vision numbness or tingling in the feet or hands wounds that do not heal unexplained weight loss

Symptoms of type 2 diabetes generally develop slowly—over the course of many years—and might be so minor that you might not even notice them. Many folks have no symptoms. Some individuals may not discover they have the condition until they develop diabetes-related health concerns, such as impaired vision or heart disease.

CAUSE OF TYPE 2 DIABETES

Type 2 diabetes , the most prevalent type of diabetes is caused by numerous causes, including lifestyle factors and genes.

1. Overweight, obesity, and physical inactivity: You are more prone to acquire type 2 diabetes if you are not physically active and are overweight or have obesity. Extra weight occasionally promotes insulin resistance and is frequent in persons with type 2 diabetes. The location of body fat also makes a difference. Extra belly fat is connected to insulin resistance, type 2 diabetes, and heart and blood vessel damage. To learn whether your weight puts you at risk for type 2 diabetes, check out these Body Mass Index (BMI) charts

2. Insulin resistance: Type 2 diabetes generally starts with insulin resistance, a condition in which muscle, liver, and fat cells do not utilize insulin properly. As a consequence, your body requires extra insulin to help glucose enter cells. Initially, the pancreas manufactures

extra insulin to keep up with the additional demand. Over time, the pancreas can't create enough insulin, and blood glucose levels increase.

3. Genes and family history.

In type 1 diabetes, some genes may make you more susceptible to acquire type 2 diabetes. The illness tends to run in families and occurs more commonly in following racial/ethnic groups:

African Americans
Alaska Natives
American Indians
Asian Americans
Hispanics/Latinos
Native Hawaiians Pacific Islanders

Genes also may raise the risk of type 2 diabetes by raising a person's inclination to become overweight or develop obesity.

RISK FACTORS THAT LEAD TO TYPE 2 DIABETES

Type 2 diabetes is partially a hereditary illness and partly a lifestyle disorder. People whose parents had diabetes have a genetic tendency, meaning they are more likely to have type 2 diabetes themselves. While there is no one reason for acquiring Type 2 diabetes, there are well-known risk factors. others of them can be modified (avoidable) and others cannot (unavoidable).

UNAVOIDABLE RISK FACTOR

The family history of diabetes — those with close relatives who have type 2 diabetes are more likely to have the ailment themselves. Moreover one in ten of individuals with a sibling who has type 2 diabetes will get the illness, as will half of those with an identical twin who is plagued by type 2 diabetes.

- Age - the danger rises as a person grows older.
- Ethnic background - persons from Aboriginal or Torres Strait Islanders, Pacific Islanders, Indian and Chinese ethnic background are more prone to acquire type 2 diabetes mellitus.
- Having Polycystic Ovarian Syndrome or a history of gestational diabetes during pregnancy.
- Low birth weight is considered to predispose to diabetes owing to poor beta-cell formation and function.

AVOIDABLE RISK FACTORS

- Obesity and overweight
- Physical inactivity
- High blood pressure Diet
- Impaired glucose metabolism

COMPLICATIONS OF TYPE 2 DIABETES

The elevated blood glucose found in diabetes may damage blood vessels, neurons, and organs, leading to a range of possible problems. Some instances of the problems produced by diabetes include the following:

- Heart Disease and Stroke: A persistently high blood glucose level may raise the risk of blood arteries getting constricted and blocked with fatty plaques (atherosclerosis). This may alter blood flow to the heart producing angina and in rare circumstances, heart attack. If blood arteries that supply the brain are damaged, this may lead to stroke.
- Nervous System Damage: Excess hyperglycemia in the blood may damage tiny blood vessels in the nerves generating a tingling feeling or discomfort in the fingers, toes, and

limbs. Nerves that are outside of the central nervous system may also be injured, which is referred to as peripheral neuropathy. If nerves of the gastrointestinal system are damaged, this may induce vomiting, constipation, and diarrhea.

- Diabetic Retinopathy: Damage to the retina may occur if small vessels in this layer of tissue get clogged or start to leak. A light then fails to pass through the retina adequately which might cause visual loss.
- Kidney Disease: Blockage and leaking of vessels in the kidneys may compromise renal function. This generally arises as a consequence of high blood pressure and blood pressure control is an essential element of treating type 2 diabetes.
- Foot Ulceration: Nerve loss in the feet might mean tiny injuries are not felt or addressed, which can lead to a foot

ulcer forming. This occurs to roughly 10% of persons with diabetes.

DIAGNOSIS AND TREATMENT

Type 2 diabetes mellitus is diagnosed when any of the following criteria are reached:

1. Symptoms of diabetes are present (increased urination, increased thirst or weight loss) with a random plasma glucose (RPG) level of >11.0mmol/L
2. Fasting plasma glucose (FPG) >7.0mmol/L
3. Oral glucose tolerance test (OGTT) 2-hour plasma glucose >11.1mmol/L

Patients who do not reach these criteria may still be classified as having impaired fasting glucose (IFG) or impaired glucose tolerance (IGT) on the basis of fasting blood glucose or oral glucose tolerance test results. These patients are at increased risk of developing type 2 diabetes mellitus.

PREVENTION OF TYPE 2 DIABETES .

Healthy lifestyle choices can help prevent type 2 diabetes, and that's true even if you have diabetes in your family. If you've already received a diagnosis of diabetes, you can use healthy lifestyle choices to help prevent complications. If you have prediabetes, lifestyle changes can slow or stop the progression of diabetes.

A healthy lifestyle includes:

- Eating healthy foods. Choose foods lower in fat and calories and higher in fiber. Focus on fruits, vegetables, and whole grains.
- Getting active. Aim for a minimum of 30 to 60 minutes of moderate physical activity — or 15 to 30 minutes of vigorous aerobic activity — on most

days. Take a brisk daily walk. Ride a bike. Swim laps. If you can't fit in a long workout, spread your activity throughout the day.

- Losing weight. If you're overweight, losing 5 to 10 percent of your body weight can reduce the risk of diabetes. To keep your weight in a healthy range, focus on permanent changes to your eating and exercise habits. Motivate yourself by remembering the benefits of losing weight, such as a healthier heart, more energy, and improved self-esteem.
- Avoiding being sedentary for long periods. Sitting still for long periods can increase your risk of type 2 diabetes. Try to get up every 30 minutes and move around for at least a few minutes.
- Sometimes medication is an option as well. Metformin (Glucophage, Glumetza, others), an oral diabetes medication, may reduce the risk of

type 2 diabetes. But even if you take medication, healthy lifestyle choices remain essential for preventing or managing diabetes.

CHAPTER FOUR

PREDIABETES

Prediabetes happens when you have elevated blood sugar levels, but they're not high enough to be considered Type 2 diabetes.

Healthy blood sugar (glucose) levels are 70 to 99 milligrams per deciliter (mg/dL). If you have undiagnosed prediabetes, your levels are typically 100 to 125 mg/dL.

According to the American Diabetes Association, for people 45 years old with prediabetes, the 10-year risk of developing Type 2 diabetes is 9% to 14%. The good news is that it's possible to reverse prediabetes with healthy lifestyle changes.

Prediabetes is very common. Researchers estimate that 84 million adults in the U.S. have prediabetes. It affects more than 1 in 3 adults under age 65 and half of people over 65 in the U.S.

More than 80% of people with prediabetes don't know they have it, as it often has no symptoms.

SYMPTOMS OF PREDIABETES

Most people with prediabetes don't have any symptoms. This is why it's important to see your primary care provider regularly so they can do screenings, like a basic metabolic panel, to check on your blood sugar levels. This is the only way to know if you have prediabetes.

For the few people who do experience symptoms of prediabetes, they may include:

- Darkened skin in your armpit or back and sides of your neck (acanthosis nigricans).
- Skin tags.

- Eye changes that can lead to diabetes-related retinopathy.

CAUSE OF PREDIABETES

The cause of prediabetes is mainly insulin resistance.

Insulin resistance happens when cells in your muscles, fat and liver don't respond as they should to insulin. Insulin is a hormone your pancreas makes that's essential for life and regulating blood sugar levels. When you don't have enough insulin or your body doesn't respond properly to it, you experience elevated blood sugar levels.

Several factors can contribute to insulin resistance, including:

- Genetics.

- Excess body fat, especially in your belly and around your organs (visceral fat).
- Physical inactivity.
- Eating highly processed, high-carbohydrate foods and saturated fats frequently.
- Certain medications, like long-term steroid use.
- Hormonal disorders, like hypothyroidism and Cushing syndrome.
- Chronic stress and a lack of quality sleep.

RISK FACTORS FOR PREDIABETES

Risk factors for prediabetes include:

- Family history of Type 2 diabetes (parent or sibling).
- Having overweight or obesity (a BMI greater than 25).

- Being physically active fewer than three times a week.
- Smoking.
- Obstructive sleep apnea.
- Having had gestational diabetes.
- Polycystic ovarian syndrome (PCOS).

Race and ethnicity are also factors. You're at increased risk if you are:
Black.
Hispanic/Latino American.
Native American.
Pacific Islander.
Asian American.

Some of these risk factors you can't change, like your age and family history (genetics). But others, like physical inactivity and smoking, you can help improve. The more of these risk factors you have, the more likely prediabetes is around the corner — or you already have it.

It's important to talk to your primary care provider about screening for prediabetes. While it might be mentally easier to avoid finding out, knowing and taking action are very valuable to your long-term health.

POSSIBLE COMPLICATIONS OF PREDIABETES

The main complication of prediabetes is it developing into Type 2 diabetes. Undiagnosed or undermanaged Type 2 diabetes increases your risk of several complications, like:

- Heart attack and stroke.
- Eye issues (diabetes-related retinopathy).
- Kidney issues (diabetes-related nephropathy).
- Nerve damage (diabetes-related neuropathy).

is it possible to reverse prediabetes? , it's typically not possible to reverse diabetes complications. This is why prevention and/or proper management are key.

DIAGNOSIS AND TEST

Healthcare providers rely on routine blood test screenings to check for prediabetes. If you have risk factors for prediabetes, your provider may recommend these screenings more often.

The following tests can check for prediabetes:

1. Fasting plasma glucose test: This tests your blood after you haven't had anything to eat or drink except water for at least eight hours beforehand (fasted). Basic metabolic panels and comprehensive metabolic panels include a glucose test. Providers

routinely order these to get an overall look at your health.

2. A1C test: This test provides your average blood glucose level over the past two to three months.

Your provider would diagnose you with prediabetes if your:

- Fasting plasma glucose test result is 100 to 125 mg/dL (normal is less than 100; diabetes is 126 or higher).
- A1C result is 5.7% to 6.4% (normal is less than 5.7%; diabetes is 6.5% or higher).

MANAGEMENT AND TREATMENT OF PREDIABETES

The best way to treat — and potentially reverse — prediabetes is through healthy lifestyle changes. Regularly eating nutritious foods and getting regular exercise can help return your blood sugar to healthy levels and prevent or delay Type 2 diabetes.

Even small changes can significantly lower your risk for developing Type 2 diabetes, like:

- Weight loss: Your healthcare provider may recommend trying to lose excess weight to combat insulin resistance and prediabetes. One study revealed that losing 7% of weight can reduce the onset of Type 2 diabetes by 58%.
- Regular activity: Getting regular amounts of moderate-intensity physical activity helps increase glucose usage and improve muscle insulin sensitivity. A single session of moderate-intensity exercise can increase glucose uptake from your blood and into your muscles by at least 40%. This helps lower blood sugar levels. Aim for 30 minutes a day, five days a week, for a total of 150

minutes a week. Try walking or another activity you enjoy.

- Eating changes: Cutting out added sugars, swapping simple carbohydrates for complex carbohydrates and eating more veggies can help your blood sugar return to healthy levels. Your provider will help you find which long-term diet for prediabetes is best for you.

Lowering your risk factors for prediabetes can often get your blood sugar levels back to healthy levels. You might:

- Work with a nutritionist or dietitian to plan healthy eating patterns you can stick with long-term, like the Mediterranean diet.
- Find ways to reduce or manage stress.
- Quit smoking.
- Get a diagnosis for and/or treat any sleep disorders.
- Manage related conditions, like high cholesterol and high blood pressure.

- Find support groups where you can meet other people going through the same challenges.

There are many programs available to help people live healthy lives and reverse prediabetes. To find a plan that works for you, talk to your provider or find resources through the National Diabetes Prevention Program.

In some cases, your healthcare provider may recommend taking certain oral diabetes medications. This is more likely if lifestyle changes haven't helped improve your blood sugar levels and/or you have multiple risk factors for Type 2 diabetes.

The most common medications providers prescribe for prediabetes are metformin and acarbose.

PREVENTION OF PREDIABETES

The strategies for preventing prediabetes are the same as for reversing it and preventing Type 2 diabetes:

- Exercising regularly.
- Maintaining a weight that's healthy for you.
- Eating nutritious food.
- Not smoking.

Unfortunately, some people have such strong genetic risk factors that even lifestyle changes aren't enough to prevent developing prediabetes.

OUTLOOK /PROGNOSIS

What can I expect if I have prediabetes?
If you receive a prediabetes diagnosis, you'll need to make lifestyle changes to manage or reverse it. This can be overwhelming. But taking it one step at a time can lead you closer to better health.

Without taking action, many people with prediabetes eventually develop Type 2 diabetes. This is often because people don't know they have prediabetes.

HOW TO TAKE CARE OF YOURSELF IF YOU ARE DIAGNOSED WITH PREDIABETES

Aside from following your healthcare team's medical guidance for treating prediabetes, there are other things you can do to help make life with prediabetes a little easier, including:

- Educate yourself: Diabetes is complex, and many things affect blood sugar levels. Do your best to educate yourself on prediabetes and diabetes from reliable sources. And don't hesitate to ask your healthcare provider questions.

- Educate family and friends: The more your loved ones know about prediabetes and the changes you're making to help your health, the more they can support you in this journey.
- Take care of your mental health: A prediabetes diagnosis can make you feel all sorts of emotions, especially because of the widespread stigma and misunderstanding about diabetes. If prediabetes is causing you distress, consider seeing a mental health professional, like a psychologist.

It's also important to remember:

- Changing habits is difficult. It likely won't be a straightforward path to healthier habits. This is OK and expected.
- Focus on one goal or healthy change at a time. Too many changes at once can be overwhelming.

- Value progress over perfection. Any positive change is a helpful change.
- Be kind to yourself.

If you still develop prediabetes or Type 2 diabetes despite making healthy changes, try not to be hard on yourself. Type 2 diabetes isn't a disease of a lack of willpower. It involves many complex mechanisms. And the healthy changes you've made are still helping protect your health.

It's important to see your healthcare provider regularly if you have prediabetes or are at increased risk for it. Even if your management plan is currently working, your needs and body may change. So, it's important to check in with your provider consistently. They'll let you know how frequently to have appointments.

What questions should I ask my healthcare provider about prediabetes?

It can be helpful to ask these questions:

- How can I lower my risk for prediabetes and Type 2 diabetes
- What are the symptoms of Type 2 diabetes?
- What's a healthy and realistic weight for me to aim for?
- What are some healthy ways to lose weight and keep it off?
- How much physical activity should I do and what kind is best for me?
- What changes can I make to my eating patterns to help prevent or delay Type 2 diabetes?
- Should I see a registered dietitian? If so, who do you recommend?
- Can you refer me to a diabetes prevention program nearby or online?
- Are there any local support groups for people with prediabetes or diabetes?

CHAPTER FIVE

GESTATIONAL DIABETES

Gestational diabetes is a type of diabetes that can develop during pregnancy in women who don't already have diabetes. Every year, 2% to 10% of pregnancies in the United States are affected by gestational diabetes. Managing gestational diabetes will help make sure you have a healthy pregnancy and a healthy baby.

CAUSE OF GESTATIONAL DIABETES

Gestational diabetes occurs when your body can't make enough insulin during your pregnancy. Insulin is a hormone made by your pancreas that acts like a key to let blood sugar into the cells in your body for use as energy.

During pregnancy, your body makes more hormones and goes through other changes, such as weight gain. These changes cause your body's cells to use insulin less effectively, a condition called insulin resistance. Insulin resistance increases your body's need for insulin.

All pregnant women have some insulin resistance during late pregnancy. However, some women have insulin resistance even before they get pregnant. They start pregnancy with an increased need for insulin and are more likely to have gestational diabetes.

SYMPTOMS AND RISK OF GESTATIONAL DIABETES

Gestational diabetes typically doesn't have any symptoms. Your medical history and whether you have any risk factors may suggest to your doctor that you could have gestational diabetes, but you'll need to be tested to know for sure.

RELATED HEALTH PROBLEMS .

Having gestational diabetes can increase your risk of high blood pressure during pregnancy. It can also increase your risk of having a large baby that needs to be delivered by cesarean section (C-section).

If you have gestational diabetes, your baby is at higher risk of:

- Being very large (9 pounds or more), which can make delivery more difficult
- Being born early, which can cause breathing and other problems
- Having low blood sugar
- Developing type 2 diabetes later in life

Your blood sugar levels will usually return to normal after your baby is born. However, about 50% of women with gestational diabetes go on to develop type 2 diabetes. You can lower your risk by reaching a healthy body weight after delivery. Visit your doctor to have your blood sugar tested 6 to 12 weeks after your baby is born and then every 1 to 3 years to make sure your levels are on target.

TEST FOR GESTATIONAL DIABETES

It's important to be tested for gestational diabetes so you can begin treatment to protect your health and your baby's health.

Gestational diabetes usually develops around the 24th week of pregnancy, so you'll probably be tested between 24 and 28 weeks.

If you're at higher risk for gestational diabetes, your doctor may test you earlier. Blood sugar that's higher than normal early in your pregnancy may indicate you have type 1 or type 2 diabetes rather than gestational diabetes.

PREVENTION OF GESTATIONAL DIABETES

Before you get pregnant, you may be able to prevent gestational diabetes by losing weight if you're overweight and getting regular physical activity.

Don't try to lose weight if you're already pregnant. You'll need to gain some weight—but not too quickly—for your baby to be healthy. Talk to your doctor about how much weight you should gain for a healthy pregnancy.

TREATMENT FOR GESTATIONAL DIABETES

You can do a lot to manage your gestational diabetes. Go to all your prenatal

in your pregnancy may indicate you have
type 1 or type 2 diabetes rather than
gestational diabetes.

PREVENTION OF GESTATIONAL DIABETES

Before you get pregnant, you may be able to
prevent gestational diabetes by losing
weight if you're overweight and getting
regular physical activity.

Don't try to lose weight if you're already
pregnant. You'll need to gain some
weight—but not too quickly—for your baby
to be healthy. Talk to your doctor about how
much weight you should gain for a healthy
pregnancy.

TREATMENT FOR GESTATIONAL DIABETES

You can do a lot to manage your gestational
diabetes. Go to all your prenatal

diabetes go on to develop type 2 diabetes. You can lower your risk by reaching a healthy body weight after delivery. Visit your doctor to have your blood sugar tested 6 to 12 weeks after your baby is born and then every 1 to 3 years to make sure your levels are on target.

TEST FOR GESTATIONAL DIABETES

It's important to be tested for gestational diabetes so you can begin treatment to protect your health and your baby's health.

Gestational diabetes usually develops around the 24th week of pregnancy, so you'll probably be tested between 24 and 28 weeks.

If you're at higher risk for gestational diabetes, your doctor may test you earlier. Blood sugar that's higher than normal early appointments and follow your treatment plan, including:

- Checking your blood sugar to make sure your levels stay in a healthy range.
- Eating healthy food in the right amounts at the right times. Follow a healthy eating plan created by your doctor or dietitian.
- Being active. Regular physical activity that's moderately intense (such as brisk walking) lowers your blood sugar and makes you more sensitive to insulin so your body won't need as much. Make sure to check with your doctor about what kind of physical activity you can do and if there are any kinds you should avoid.
- Monitoring your baby. Your doctor will check your baby's growth and development.

If healthy eating and being active aren't enough to manage your blood sugar, your doctor may prescribe insulin, metformin, or other medication.